WE ARE NOT DONE

by

Linda Alexander

CONTENTS

Dedication & Acknowledgements..........................1

Foreword 3

Introduction 6

So, What's YOUR Story?.................................15

The Mindset 28

Purpose and Goals 38

Stress..55

Support..65

Training 72

Nutrition 91

Lifestyle 104

Bonus Materials 113

About the Author 123

Dedication & Acknowledgements

This book is dedicated to my family, my inner circle, those related by blood and by love. Their endless support, and guidance have helped me truly become my best self.

Thank you to those who have helped me create this book.

My three girls for standing by me and always supporting me.

My mom Jeri and my sisters, Kathi and Renee for their unconditional love and support.

Mandi Love for her support, encouragement, and help throughout this entire project and for helping me make it pretty.

My clients who inspire me every day to be a better coach.

Pat Rigsby for gently pushing me to start this project, and his continual support.

Kerri Nelson, my editor, for her guidance, patience and encouragement.

Ethan Harper for his beautiful butterfly drawing.

Foreword

I first met Linda in 2010 when I walked through the door of her studio as a client.

Two years earlier, I had suffered the sudden loss of my father and subsequently found myself struggling to balance everyday life for myself and for my family.

I was constantly putting everyone and everything before my own health, leaving me feeling mentally, emotionally and physically exhausted.

I wanted to make healthy changes, but I didn't know how. I had no direction.

I knew, with the right support and program, that I would be able to make those changes and begin to feel stronger again.

I had finally found the right coach.

Linda understood my struggle and knew exactly what I needed to do to reach my fitness goals.

I followed the tools found in this book, trusted the process, made gradual changes, and began to live a healthier, more balanced life.

The information Linda is going to share with you is so important because she helps you understand a different way at looking at your approach to your health, your fitness, your life, and yourself.

Her book is a step by step guide to incorporating realistic practices into one's every day hectic schedule, that maybe had once seemed to be overwhelming.

For me, making these changes saved my life.

Linda understands struggle. She understands all the balancing acts, stresses, and demands that, as women, we place on ourselves. She brings this personal experience, combined with her expertise, to have developed an unparalleled program.

She celebrates each and every achievement, no matter how big or how small. She is committed to being a source of encouragement and support for any individual who is trying to better their health.

Linda's coaching experience, as well as her passion in providing guidance and support, will undoubtedly help you find a healthy balance towards becoming your best self.

This is what sets her apart from anyone I have ever met.

I have always been, and will forever remain, incredibly thankful and proud of the person she is.

Mandi Love, NASM CPT
Spartan Specialist

Introduction

If you were standing in front of me, you would probably say "how can she relate to me about losing weight when she clearly doesn't need to lose any herself?" True, I have not gone through a WEIGHT transformation, however I have gone through many other transformations in my lifetime. And being a good coach means helping others reach their potential, no matter what the fine details are. Coaching is coaching. Good coaches will rely on their own personal experiences to help create the right strategies for their clients. I have learned that one of the things that connects us as women, and as human beings, is that we all struggle with something at various points in our lives. We all need guidance and support at times, and it often has nothing to do with weight. I am sharing my story with you in the hopes that understanding more about my challenges, you will trust that I am the right coach to guide you on your own healthy lifestyle transformation.

As a child I was constantly on the go, spending most of my time outdoors. As I got older, I started playing organized sports and found that I was pretty good at them. Most athletics I chose came pretty easily to me. I felt most comfortable either playing sports or being outside. I had found my wheelhouse, or my safe place-- the one place where I felt good at something!

After I graduated college and got married, I continued to be active in sports, even taking up new ones to keep the fire inside me alive. I coached high school volleyball and played volleyball on several different teams. I learned to play golf and I took up tennis. The success and love I found in tennis, created a path towards becoming a teaching tennis pro. Again I found my wheelhouse, my safe place, this time both playing and coaching.

Fast forward a few years, three amazing girls and three major moves, one to a different country, and I land in Richmond, Virginia. I was living in a new city with the "perfect" family, the "perfect" house and the "perfect" life. From the outside world's perspective, I had it all. But on the inside I was dying. I was living a lie and I was completely unhappy. Something needed to change and I knew I was not being my best self.

My personal transformation began, as it does with many people, with a dramatic change in my lifestyle. For me, it was a divorce, but after my divorce, I went right to my safe place - MOVEMENT. I started a very unhealthy training program, which consisted of being in the gym for two hours or more a day, trying just to feel better. My physical body changed, but my mind didn't. My wheelhouse was letting me down! Again, I looked great on the outside, and from the outside world's perspective, it was, wow she looks great! But on the inside I was still dying, and NOT being my best self. My whole self was not healthy and I knew I had to change more in order to feed my whole self.

Fast forward again a few more years, a few failed relationships, and the feeling my daughters are growing up WAY TOO FAST, I needed a plan that would make me whole. I again went back to my wheelhouse. I needed to MOVE. I was no longer teaching tennis and was strictly coaching fitness. Then it clicked, I realized that many of my clients were women just like me, wanting more for themselves, wanting to be whole. I knew I could help them physically because THAT was what I was good at. I was a great coach and knew that I could get them where they wanted to be physically. At the time I was working at one of the local gyms in the area, and realized our training philosophies were drastically different. So, that's when I decided to open my own studio! Oxygen and Iron Personal Training Studio. Which was amazing, for many reasons. I was finally able to decide what was best for my clients, instead of a corporation's opinion. I started with a business partner and we worked long hours to get it open and thriving.

Fast forward 5 years, and the business partnership was not working out as expected. We had different visions for the studio and we needed to part ways. Time for another change! After many months of debating what would be the right thing to do, I decided to take over sole ownership of the studio. Now I'm standing in a studio alone, my first thought is Oh crap, what I have I gotten myself into? but after the fear subsided a bit, I got excited and thought Oh crap look what I can create with this place! I built my own WHEELHOUSE!

The studio was doing great. I was building my ideal business. Running a business is more than coaching clients, it's more than writing training programs and helping with nutrition. There are many behind the scenes projects that only a business owner would understand. This I didn't realize until it was coming down to just me to get everything done. I had to learn how to continue to be a great coach, but also be a great business owner! So, I needed a coach as well. Once I found the perfect one for my business goals, plus the help from my fantastic staff of coaches, things started to fall into place. Am I where I want to be on my business? NO. But I continue to learn and get better every year, every day.

My business continued to thrive and I was finally enjoying the rhythm between helping my clients succeed and balancing the demands of the business. But then, as the theme is, life threw me another curveball. My dad's health began to deteriorate over the summer. The person who taught me how to be an athlete and how to play-- his body was failing him. I spent several months flying back and forth from Virginia to Florida to spend time with him, and to support my mom who was his 24/7 nurse and caregiver. We lost my dad in December 2015. Life now has forever changed for my whole family. The months following his death were both foggy and uncomfortable, I was seeking my new normal.

To get back on track, I focused on my much needed training program again, the one I had let slack because of lack of time and lack of desire. But this time was a little different. I was going to coach myself like one of my own clients. So, I wrote my goals and I got myself a coach, hoping that would help keep me on track. I decided to try my first Spartan race. Spartan race is an obstacle course race, ranging from 3-12+ or so miles with around 25+ obstacles thrown in throughout the course. The Virginia Spartan Race was on a mountain that particular year.

I thought that would be a good way to get me focused both mentally and physically. Well, it did the trick. I had a pretty good race for my first one and being over 50 years old, it was a good but demanding challenge. I had trained hard and it payed off on race day! My two main goals of my first OCR race were, to finish and to not to get hurt! I accomplished both and was excited enough to start training for my next one!

The race was in September of 2016. The next month, I went in for a regular checkup and was told I needed an echocardiogram for my heart murmur. REALLY? I had always known I had a heart murmur and it never was a concern of mine. I was healthy, active, and I trained almost every day, I ate well, and most of all I felt great! But, the echogram didn't go as well as expected. I was told I needed heart valve surgery. HEART SURGERY? Really? But, I felt great! No symptoms of a supposedly bad heart. Plus, I just finished a Spartan Race, in the mountains, how could I possibly have a bad heart? Again, another curveball. So, I found the best surgeon in Richmond and he performed the surgery flawlessly. I was out of the hospital in 4 days and I went back to work after 2 months. Never did I believe that I would have heart surgery. However, I learned that even when you do everything right to be healthy, sometimes you don't get to choose your outcome.

Today, I have realized that helping women become their best self is NOT just about how they look, or about their nutrition plan, it's more about creating their whole self and what it takes to get there, one step at a time. Through my own challenges and transformations, I have become a better coach. I can see where these women can become stuck in their same old ways, and how I am better prepared to guide them.

I still have women say to me when they first meet me, how can you relate to me about WEIGHT loss when you don't look like you need to lose any weight? I'm guessing that will never change. Though I won't go through the entire history of me, I can tell them how I relate to the feeling of wanting to change. The fears, the hopes, the wanting of a better self. I remind them that no matter how healthy you are, even if you do everything right, sometimes you don't get to choose your outcome. Sometimes the curveballs choose you. You do, however, have the choice to make yourself healthier on the inside and out, but you may need a little help and guidance.

We Are Not Done.

1

So, What's YOUR Story?

Do you miss that strong healthy woman you used to be? You remember a time when you felt invincible. You could eat what you wanted. You had the stamina to go all day long. You were carefree.

Somewhere along the way, you lost some of that confidence, that strength, and vigor. I know how it feels, but it's time for you to make a change, because you deserve to enjoy your life and become your best self. It doesn't matter if you are in your 30's, 40's, 50's or older, you can live a healthier lifestyle. It truly is never too late to start!

We all strive to be our best self, to be healthy, workout and eat right. We know it's good for us, and the right thing to do. So, why is it so hard to get started or stick with it?

Let's follow three women and discover how they made a few changes in their lives to become the best versions of themselves. With a little guidance of course.

Let's meet the ladies:

Jennifer, a real go getter, in her mid-30's and thought she was pretty healthy. She goes to the gym every day, but her plan or lack of plan was not working for her.

Ann, in her late 40's, married with three kids, and some days feels like a taxi driver. Claims she doesn't have time to be healthy, but really she has never been someone who works out and is a little intimidated walking into a gym.

Susan, empty nester, with lots of free time, ready to enjoy her grandkids and is worried she won't be able to keep up with them.

Three different women at different stages in their lives, but all looking to feel better, move better and live better. Find out how following a few simple guidelines, helped get them on the path to living a healthier lifestyle and becoming their best selves.

You have many factors that determine if you are living a healthy life. For example, do you workout, eat healthy foods, know how to manage your stress? What you do every day decides if you are healthy or you need some help. Health is a choice. It doesn't just happen. You actually get to choose what you put in your mouths, if you move your body and how you think.

Most of us start out healthy as babies, your body is able to move freely and you have no mental worries. But however, as you age, most of those traits start to deteriorate. Again, by the choices you make. Your habits and actions directly affect how you look, feel and move. As well as the quality of the life in your later years. But, it's not too late! You can get that vigor back and feel like a kid again! It's about making smart choices.

So, how do you get healthy?

The first step is knowing that you want or need to change to make yourself healthy. You change because you want something or because you are afraid you will lose something. Becoming your best self takes work, dedication and support.

Is it going to be easy? No!

Is it going to be worth it? ABSOLUTELY YES!

The number one reason most women initially come to see us is that they think they need help in achieving weight loss. After we start working together, we find that weight is actually a symptom and often not the reason at all.

What you really need is guidance, structure, and accountability. You are looking for someone that's going to give you a plan to feeling better, both mentally and physically, while helping you achieve your health and fitness goals. Women, like yourself, need someone who understands you, listens to you, and someone who has been in your shoes.

We will discuss some of the biggest challenges for most women in the chapters ahead, and look inside three of our members who have overcome some of these challenges.

One of the most common complaints we hear is, "I'm too busy, how could I possibly find any time in my schedule for me and my goals?" The simple truth is that we are all busy, we are all over extended and have way too much on our plates. But I'm here to tell you, it can be done. You see, if it is truly important enough to you,

you will find time to do it. You find the time to have dinner with friends, to keep work meetings, family commitments, and even to get your hair done.

You just need to look at aspects of your health as that important and just make time for it. I know you are probably thinking, that's easy for me to say, but I help women change their lives every day. If you simply make a few small changes, or tweaks to your current lifestyle, you will be amazed how much time you can find, how much better you look and feel and best of all, you will become the BEST version of you. Plus, you will also be the BEST version of you for your loved ones as well.

Maybe you are a woman who has found the time to eat healthy and exercise, but still can't seem to lose the weight you want or get the strength you desire. You may be a gym rat, a runner or a long time "yo-yo" dieter.

Or are you, the woman who has never exercised? You never understood how to exercise properly and feel insecure walking into a gym. You want to be healthy but don't know where to start. And, quite frankly, your life is chaotic with children and everyday errands.

Lastly, you might be someone who has the time and your desired weight, but are worried about your mobility and strength as you grow older? You are in the prime of your life with no children living at home anymore, more free time to travel and start new hobbies. But, you also worry that it's the time of more medical problems. Such as, the need for possible blood pressure and cholesterol medications, or pending joint replacements. You want to stay healthy and active for your grandchildren and your new adventures.

Throughout this book we are going to breakdown the plans these three ladies used and help find the ones you may need to live a healthy lifestyle. We will keep it simple, to help you see real success. And it's not just about the workouts or eating chicken and broccoli!

It will be proven tips, hacks, and solutions I have used for over 30 years, to guide you to a new healthier YOU!

What you won't find in this book are boring and difficult to interpret facts with scientific calculations regarding exercise and nutrition. Our goal is to provide you with a simple plan that is relatable. We make it simple so you can understand the steps you need in order to be successful. All of our information is scientific and factual. However, we want to equip you with tools, not statistics. Empower you with a plan, not bore you to death with the science. If you want to know more about the science, I know someone named Google.

We have identified seven areas that will help guide you on your path to success. The 7 steps helpful to live a healthy balanced enjoyable life!

Mindset
Stress Management
Support and Recovery
Purpose and Goals

Exercise
Nutrition
Lifestyle

In the following chapters, we will explain why you need to work on your current habits, which are at this stage, comfortable, and create new habits in each area and which action steps to take in order to become your new future self. I understand change is hard, but if you break down these new habits into small action steps it will make the process easier and longer lasting. In addition, you will learn from our three ladies how they used these strategies to live their healthiest lives, it's time to meet the ladies whose lives have changed for the better...

JENNIFER:

Goes to the gym day after day, doing the same thing. Treadmill first, next some weight machines and then maybe hit the elliptical for the last 30 minutes. She feels like she is eating right, but may have an occasional glass of wine or two at dinner. Her Fitbit tells her that she has walked over 10,000 steps today, but she just can't seem to lose the weight. Even worse, she is constantly tired all the time and has to keep buying the next size up. Jennifer wonders: "This whole exercise and eating right is hard, and what's the point when you see no results?"

ANN:

It's 2:30 and the kids are almost finished with school. Ann has been up for hours and has been going non-stop since about 5:30 am. Already she has packed lunches, made beds, gone grocery shopping, dropped off her youngest son's homework that he forgot at school, and she is still only half way down her to do list. Ann didn't have breakfast except for the latte and the "healthy muffin" she picked up at the drive-thru. She is starving, cranky and feels like she just got hit by a truck. Yet, she powers through, because the boys have soccer practice and her daughter has a guitar lesson after school. So she grabs another latte and picks up her kids. After all the after school activities are through and she and her family have finished dinner, it's time for homework, baths and bedtime and then finally Ann sits down to relax. Feeling exhausted and stiff. Ann wonders: "How has my life become so chaotic?" Ann knows she needs to live a healthier life, one for herself, but also to be a good role model for her children. But honestly, Ann is afraid to join a gym, she has visions of only healthy fit people all wearing tight fitting clothing and looking beautiful. If she actually found the courage to step into a gym, she has no clue what to do when she gets there. With all different equipment, it's intimidating, she doesn't want to look foolish or hurt herself.

SUSAN:

Now that the kids are out of the house completely, she has more free time to do as she pleases. It has been that way for a few years now, since the kids started driving for themselves and then away at college. Susan has been feeling this shift coming for years. It is now time to take care of herself, it's "me time." But what she has found, by not taking care of herself properly over the past few years is that it has caused her to lose some strength and balance. Her knees hurt going up the stairs and her back is sore when she sits too long. She knows it won't be long before she retires and grandchildren will be on their way at some point. Susan wants to be active for them as well as herself, plus she sees many of her friends getting knee and hip replacements and she knows she doesn't want to go down that road. She too is nervous about walking into a gym, because those same friends have told her horror stories about the trainers (not coaches) they have used in the past.

Can you picture yourself in any or part of these women?

Most of us can relate to all or at least part of their stories, stories like these come through our doors every day.

Now it's your turn to discover your best self.

It's time to uncover that strength you never knew you had, but could develop with the right guidance and support. Get your stamina back and have more confidence. Now is the time you can take control of your life and become your best self.

You can do it!

I know you can.

I watch the magic of women changing their lives for the better every day. All you needed was a guide, and it would be my pleasure to help you become your best self!

2

The Mindset

Even though this book is about how to live a healthier lifestyle, you may have noticed I did not start with exercise or nutrition. As important as they are, other areas stand out first and will have a much greater impact on getting you to a healthier lifestyle. The one I feel is most important is Mindset and that is why we start here first.

What is Mindset? Why is it so important?

Mindset is simply our beliefs and thoughts we have about ourselves and how we handle our thoughts in different situations. The body will only do what the mind tells it to do. In other words, your actions are controlled by your mind, so, if you tell yourself that you can't lose weight, your subconscious mind will find ways to sabotage your weight loss efforts. What you tell yourself—whether it's real or not—the subconscious mind takes it as the truth. It cannot decipher between reality and fiction. If you continue to tell yourself you can't lose weight, it's too hard, well, you won't.

Remember Jennifer?

She kept telling herself that it was too hard and that she couldn't get the results she was looking for, no matter how many hours she spent in the gym or how well she ate. She asked herself: What's the point?

And Ann?

She was driving around town all day and couldn't find time to workout or eat healthy.

Both of these women had preconceived negative thoughts about training, nutrition and healthy living. But after a few small tweaks, they discovered the power of being positive and using healthy self-talk. They both decide it was time to change. Thus, the beginning of their positive mindset.

Sure you can power through life with an attitude of defeat and negative thinking and still see results of a good training program and eating a whole food diet, but this method will be hard to maintain long term.

Don't you want to live your entire life healthy and happy? Then let's start with positive self-talking.

This is the way you speak to yourselves, both verbally and non-verbally. Back to what our subconscious thinks, if you constantly tell yourself you don't have time, you can't lose weight or you are too old to train, your brain will conduct your actions to do exactly what you are telling your brain to do. You won't find time in your schedule to be healthy, you won't lose weight, because you will continue to sabotage your nutrition and you won't start a training program because you are too scared to find the right coach.

Here is a small trick we use with our clients to improve positive self-talk. Speak to yourself like you are speaking to your child, your best friend or your mom. You would kindly tell them that you are only as young as you feel and you can start a training program at any age. That you can lose weight if you find the right program and have some support. You would also tell them that you can get healthy and find the time, because you are worthy of a healthy lifestyle.

If you can just change the dialogue you tell yourself or think about yourself, you will be amazed at the impact it will have on your journey. Be kind to yourself.

YOU ARE WORTH IT.

That brings us to having a positive mindset. Thinking and speaking kindly to ourselves is a great start. Now, let's find some ways to keep your mind positive most of the time. I believe the more positive you stay, the more natural it becomes. Which, in turn, means better results and a happier you.

For me, this starts with my morning routine. I find when I stay consistent, by doing the same thing every morning, I feel better about myself and I start my day off with a Win. This is my morning routine. My daily self-care package.

MY MORNING ROUTINE:

Having a solid morning routine gets my day started with me in control of my day, not letting the day control me! First step I take when I wake up every morning is some self-care, with a big glass of water to hydrate my body and take my daily vitamins. Next come my gratitudes. I will write down three things that I am grateful for that day. This can be anything from the people in my life, to the things I am lucky enough to have in my life, or to my health and well-being. Each day is different, but I'm always grateful. We all can find at least three things we are grateful for each day. We live in a society with many things and conveniences, we have running water and a roof over our heads. Things we may take for granted each day. When you sit back and realize just how lucky you truly are, it's easy to be grateful.

I follow that up with my journal in the evening, writing again about things I am thankful for that happened that day. This is helpful to reflect on the day and realize that something good did happen today. Really put some thought behind it, don't just make it another task on your to do list that has to be checked off.

After my gratitudes, I do about 10 minutes of meditation. I have recently started this practice and have found just how helpful it has been. I am calmer during my day and when challenges come up at the studio or at home, I will stop, breathe or pause a moment, and this will help to control any negative feelings that may rise up.

Next, more self-care with my daily stretches and foam rolling to get the knots and trigger points out of my muscles. These mobility exercises keep my body limber, and most importantly gets my body ready to take on the day!

My last step is my drive into work, instead of listening to news or radio stations with mindless talking, I will use this time to listen to my favorite podcasts. Whether it's about business, training, nutrition or just learning something new, I love this time to continuously learn!

I have been giving this exact advice out to many of my clients who struggle with staying calm when under a lot of stress. Having a morning routine, will help you control how your day starts and get in the activities that are important to you. This is a giant step in helping you start your day with a positive mindset. My clients have surprisingly found it helpful too.

"When Linda told me that I should meditate, I thought she had lost her mind! One, who has 10 minutes of quiet? Two, my brain won't shut off for 1 minute, much less 10. And Three, I don't like all that tree hugger, yoga, feel good nonsense! But, I have to admit, it's starting to grow on me. I take a deep breath before snapping at the waiter who is way too slow. I find myself looking forward to the 10 minutes of not letting my brain race wild." recalled Ann, when I first introduced it to her.

I use an app called Calm (I am not an affiliate of Calm, I simply like the app). Another app I use is Headspace. Both are great. You can decide which one is best for you. Meditation is not the only tool, maybe daily prayers work better for you, what matters is you get to decide which tool works best for you!

Remember, when finding your ideal morning routine, things will come up and you won't have an ideal start every day, however if we can try to achieve most of the things in our routine, that would make our mornings smoother, and we can try and complete the rest of the morning action steps later in the day.

Another tool used at Oxygen + Iron studio is what we call the Win of the Day. It is similar to our gratitudes, but it's more of a public or private announcement of one thing that went well for us today. We use this tactic in both our in-studio and online version of our 28 Day Challenge. Each day on our private Facebook page, members post their "win of the day" each and every day. The purpose is that we rarely look at the small wins we have each day, instead we complain about what went wrong, what we didn't do and what we need to improve on. This behavior will only highlight the negative thoughts and squashes any possibility of positive self-talk. Plus, when we consistently highlight our wins, no matter how big or small, it produces a compound effect on our self-confidence, and our positive state of mind.

ACTION STEP

How is your mindset? Mostly positive? Or mostly negative? If you need a more positive mindset, try some of the tactics we discussed in this chapter. Better yet, write down your IDEAL morning routine, and make small action steps each day to get you closer to that ideal morning. Maybe you will see things looking calmer and more positive, just like Ann did.

- Positive self-talk—probably the most important factor.
- Daily gratitudes—in the morning and evening.
- Daily meditation—only 10 minutes.
- Calm app
- Headspace app
- Prayer
- Daily "Win of the Day"—take the challenge. I challenge you to try the Win of the Day, for the next 30 days, write down your win, email it to a friend, say it to your partner, heck, even post it on your Facebook page. See if it catches on with your friends.

3

Purpose and Goals

You may have tried in the past to start a new exercise or nutrition program only to fall off the wagon and go right back to your old ways. Sound familiar?

This is a common scenario for many women. You start off excited, determined and all in. Only to have something bump you off track a few weeks later. Feeling defeated, you revert back to your "old unhealthy" life again and you talk to negatively to yourself, like Jennifer did "I just can't do it, it's too hard, it doesn't work and I will always look like this!"

You tell yourself "I am too old and afraid to go to the gym" or "I am just too busy" like Susan and Ann did.

But we meet women like every day. What you don't see is that you are not alone. We help women overcome these obstacles every day. What makes them different? What gives them courage? What gives them the strength or the tenacity to change their behavior, to transform themselves into their best selves?

PURPOSE

What you need is a Purpose. We call this your WHY. What you really need is a strong WHY to get the results you are looking for.

It's time to find your Why.

This will be the MOST IMPORTANT factor in your healthy lifestyle transformation. This "why" will be different for everyone. Most importantly, it has to be YOUR reasons for transforming into the new you. YOUR personal why. No one else's. Otherwise, it just won't be strong enough to overcome the many obstacles that will be thrown your way. And kid, let me tell you, they are coming for you...obstacles, that is.

It can't come from your spouse or partner, not from your kids, or your mother. It has to be totally and completely yours. Although these very important people in our lives may be elements of your why, it all comes down to YOU.

Have I made that clear enough?

You are in charge of your destiny.

How do you find this elusive WHY? First, I'm going to ask you to time travel for just a bit.

I want you to look into the future for just a moment and imagine yourself one year from today. If you change NOTHING about your current lifestyle, what does one year from now look like to you?

How will you look?

How will you feel?

How will you live?

Now, imagine yourself taking action. You are more active, eating healthy foods, taking time for yourself, feeling less stressed and all around feeling happier about who you are.

How do you look now?

How do you feel now?

How are you living now?

I know it's hard to look into the future, because you truly can't predict it. No one can. But, if you can visualize a healthier, more active you, it helps to create the change you want.

I would never ask my members to go on some strict low fat, low carb, low calorie, crazy diet or spend hours upon hours doing mindless boring worthless cardio. Nor would I ask the same of you. Because those types of restrictions simply do not work.

What I am asking of you is to make a few changes toward your future healthy self by taking one or two habits at a time. This way you will become Your Best Self.

One step at a time with lasting results. Sounds better right?

Here is where your journey begins.

You need to find the true meaning of your why by digging deep into your answers, not superficial answers.

An example of a surface level answer is: "I need to lose a few pounds."

However, deep inside those walls you have built around your emotions and feelings of why you want to lose weight, the scary answers and feelings, the ones that have made you fail in the past. The TRUE meaning for your weight loss. That is the "why" you are looking for.

This is where it's about to get REAL!

ACTION STEP

Let's go back to the question at the beginning of this chapter. Ask yourself these two questions again, but this time get out a piece of paper or go to the back of the book and write down your answers.

If I change nothing about my lifestyle and continue on the path I am on now, what will my life look like one year from now?

How will I feel?

5 years from now?

Next, ask the second question: Now that I have learned the importance of a balanced whole food nutrition plan, I started gaining strength from my smart training program, I understood the benefits of positive self-talk, and I set aside time for me and my loved ones.

What will my life look like a year from now if I start taking care of myself?

How will these changes make me feel?

Once you have answered the second question I want you to ask yourself again, why this is important to you?

Write this down, too. Now ask yourself why again. And keep asking until you come up with the true meaning for your transformation.

For example, you may have said, "I want to lose weight."

Okay now ask, WHY do you want to lose the weight?

Your answer could be, because I want to get back down to the weight I was in college.

Why do you want to get back to that particular weight?

Because I feel I looked my best back then.

How did that make you feel looking your best?

Attractive, smart, my husband and friends noticed me more, most of all more confident.

So you want to get your confidence back and feel better about your self-esteem?

Yes, I feel like I take care of everybody else but me. Life is so busy and I have no time to get the kids where they need to go, do all my errands, or make healthy meals, there's just no time left in the day for me, let alone time for just me and my husband.

Boom!

There is the true meaning of your why. Not weight loss. Sure weight loss will be a side benefit of getting to your why, but the deep honed why is, you want more time for yourself, you want to feel confident and attractive again, you want to have your once upon a time, healthy version of you back.

Their WHY:

JENNIFER: to look better

Jennifer wanted to lose her extra weight that had been creeping on her over the past few years. With her visible "muffin top", she felt self-conscious wearing her skinny jeans, she had never had this problem in her 20's. Her 15-year class reunion was coming up. When she first came to our studio, she wanted to look stunning, but more than that she wanted to feel confident walking into that reunion with her head up high.

ANN: to feel better

Ann is busy, but knows it's important to live a healthier lifestyle. She wants to be a good role model for her children and feel better about herself both physically and mentally.

SUSAN: to move better

Susan is starting to feel the aches and pains of growing older and being sedentary most of her life. She wants to travel with her husband after they retire and she wants to be active so that she can enjoy playing with her grandchildren.

Now that you have found your true WHY, you need to eat, breathe, and live your why. This will be your cornerstone for change. Your WHY will help you stay centered and on course.

COACH'S TIP:

Here is a tip that has been proven to help many women. Having different visual cues. Writing notes to putting them on your mirror in the bathroom, or hanging on the refrigerator, so that you will see them multiple times per day. Read them out loud every time you are in front of them. Write your why on a piece of paper and keep it with you at all times, or put it as your screensaver on your computer or smartphone. Make a vision board and have it at your desk at work, or in your bedroom, so that you see it every day and you can visualize your new healthy self. This will be a constant reminder of how important your why really is. Plus, it keeps it on top of your mind every day.

It's not as easy as just writing down your why and poof! you are healthier. You will encounter obstacles. Things and people that will want to derail you from your plan. Trust me, there will be MANY roadblocks or obstacles along your journey. But first off, I want to change the dialogue in your head. It's not an obstacle or roadblock or challenge that's in your way—oh, it's something, but if you think of it as an opportunity to overcome, it won't feel as negative. Staying positive right away will allow your brain to attack it in a different way—not the end of the world way, kind of way—but something you can overcome with the right strategies. Strong Why, strong Mind and strong Body.

Don't let a weak WHY knock you off course with the first encounter!

Here are a few common challenges that may come across your path:

- Workout or weight loss plateau
- Injury or medical setback
- Fall of wagon by having one bad meal
- Vacation
- Work travel
- Special event

- Peer pressure
- Kids and Family Activities

Are your Whys strong enough to overcome all of these challenges? If not, I beg you to sit back down and dig deeper and find your strongest Why.

You need to be prepared for the journey ahead.

ACTION STEP

ROADMAP TO SUCCESS

Your journey can't start without a roadmap. A starting point with directions to follow along your course. How do you know where to start? Well, you have a great start already with your Why. Now you need a little more direction. In order to have direction, you need goals. Knowing your goals will help you take the right action steps towards living a healthier lifestyle.

Don't worry, I'm not asking you to change everything all at once. Remember this is a journey, it may take some time to become your ultimate best. But, when you develop some new healthy habits, by taking small steps at a time, I will guarantee you will look, feel and move better, one year from today.

Are you ready?

As long as you have your paper out with your why on it, let's add your goals to it. You can also find the worksheet in the back of the book.

You should have short term and long term goals. Both are needed and necessary. But in order for your goals to be most effective you need SMART goals.

A SMART goal is defined as one that is specific, measurable, achievable, results-focused, and time bound. Below is a definition of each of the S.M.A.R.T. goal criteria.

- Specific: Goals should be written simply and clearly define what you are going to do. Specific is the What, Why, and How.

- Measurable: Goals should be measurable so that you have proof that you have accomplished the goal. What gets measured, gets done!

- Achievable: Goals should be achievable; they should stretch you slightly so you feel challenged, but attainable so that you can achieve them.

- Relevant: activities that make sense with entire goal.

- Time-sensitive: Goals should be linked to a timeframe that creates a practical sense of urgency. Without such tension, the goal is unlikely to produce a relevant outcome.

To make this goal setting process easier, write down your goals according to your Why. This will keep everything aligned and your path clearer. Let's see what goal setting did for our 3 ladies.

JENNIFER: Her why: to look better for reunion and be more confident.

Her goals:

- To lose the muffin top (10 pounds) by sticking to a supportive nutrition plan.
- Train a minimum of 4 days per week until the reunion.
- Write positive notes and place them on her mirrors in the bathroom and bedroom.
- Meet up with 2 girlfriends each weekend to go hiking for at least 1 hour.

ANN: Her why: to become a good role model for her children and gain strength mentally and physically.

Her goals:
- To meditate each week for a minimum of 5 days per week.
- To start her personal training sessions once a week and group training 3 times per week.
- To start each day with a healthy breakfast which includes lean protein and vegetables.
- Take a walk with her husband and children after dinner and before homework at least 3 days per week.

SUSAN: Her why: to become more active by gaining strength and mobility and to enjoy the next chapter of her life.

Her goals:
- To start her training program with a friend and a coach 2 times per week.
- To do her mobility exercises at least 5 times per week.
- To book an active vacation at least 2 times per year with her husband.

Now that you know your why and have completed your SMART goals, you can begin to learn about what steps you need to become your best self.

4

Stress

Women are wired differently than men. We communicate differently, we have different tendencies and behaviors, our emotions work differently, we think about problems differently and we deal with stress differently.

At times, you may not recognize the level of stress you are under when it comes to everyday life. You think that just because you are multitasking, and getting things done, you are handling your stress. The truth is, you're not.

You may think that by having it all: family, career, children, friends and hobbies, makes you some type of superwoman. I am all for being a superhero (Wonder Woman would be my choice) but, chronic overload of your body and mind will only cause you problems in the long run due to stress. Also, let's not forget, that Wonder Woman is a fantasy. Nothing causes more stress than unrealistic expectations.

I remember being a single mom with 3 active girls all going in different directions at the same time. I was also trying to open my own business, while still working at a big box gym in the meantime. I got my workouts in, at least 2 hours per day and ate as healthy as I could on the go. I probably averaged 4-5 hours of sleep a night. I was tired all the time, short tempered and was getting sick more than I ever had in my past. I was miserable and knew I had to change something. What I needed to do was to learn how to manage my stress better.

One of the biggest stress makers is TIME, or what we perceive as lack of time. When you are trying to be superwoman and juggling too many things at a time, you feel like you need more hours in the day to get everything done. Time is your most finite resource you have. You can buy more stuff. Make more money and have more relationships. Basically, you can have more of anything else in life, but we are all given the same 24 hours in a day. There is no way to get one minute more. How you use your time, or manage that time, becomes a major factor on how successful you will be at living a healthy life.

JUST SAY NO

One word can help you feel happier, be less stressed and take control of your life. That word is simple, NO. Are you feeling too busy, rushed, ragged or maybe you even feel resentful for all the ways you are spending your time, saying yes to things that don't really matter, instead of actually wanting to say no.

Learn to not react to the demands of other people. Women have a natural tendency to want to be nice and please others. But, in order to get control of your precise time, you not only have the right to say no to things that don't move you towards your goals, you have the responsibility to say YES to the things that will lead you towards your success.

It's time to take responsibility for your health and well-being, and that time is now. Learn to say NO. (Politely, of course!) Then, you will be able to look at your "no" as an opportunity for someone else to say yes.

What are you willing to give up to reach your goals?

Have an honest conversation with yourself. Remember just how finite your time is and be willing to say no to less important things so that you can yes to the most important things.

Here is a great quote from Steven Covey that we can all learn from:

"Don't prioritize your schedule, schedule your priorities."

You will continue to have stress in your life. You can't avoid it. But, you can have a plan on how to manage it better. While some stress is good; like when you train, but not over-train. Exercise stresses your body for a short period of time and then it recovers.

However, when stress is bad, it not only affects your mood, it affects your entire body. Simply put, your body is not built for chronic stress.

What really happens to your body during chronic stress?

Your body releases a hormone called cortisol when it becomes stressed. Too much cortisol will elevate your blood sugar. When your blood sugar is raised, your insulin is raised, when your insulin is raised, your cortisol increases. Increased levels of cortisol cause weight gain, mostly around your belly. Do you see the vicious circle?

Most people will crave sweets when they are stressed. This is because you are depleting another hormone called serotonin. Serotonin is known as the happy hormone. When serotonin is in short supply it makes your blood sugar unstable. This will then cause you to crave more sugar. So, when you eat sugar, your blood sugar rise then falls and when it falls, you want more sugar. Another vicious cycle.

Serotonin is also the hormone that helps you sleep. When you are stressed and your Serotonin gets depleted you don't sleep well. What this means is that, some of your hormones are the culprit for weight gain, not calories. This is largely due to chronic stress.

It just keeps getting better... Just kidding. Stress is bad, really bad.

When you are stressed your stomach is at risk to get what is called leaky gut, which means it is more permeable. It makes you more intolerant to certain foods. When you have these intolerances it may start to cause inflammation in the body.

Other common side effects associated with stress (as if that weren't enough):

- Depression
- Anxiety
- Immune system dysfunctions
- Behavioral problems
- Lack of energy
- Increase blood pressure
- Decrease sex drive

Unfortunately, we all will continue to have stress in our lives. It's how you perceive that stress that matters the most. You have to learn how to manage your stress. Otherwise, there is a big price to pay.

Earlier, I explained how stressed I was when my kids were younger, and how I needed to learn how to deal with it better. Now that I am older, my stress is still there, although it may be different. However, my perspective of my stress has changed dramatically.

Today, I'm dealing with the stress of all three grown daughters, living far from home. I don't dwell on the fact that they are all out of state, rather I beam with pride knowing that they are all following their own hopes and dreams. Their aspirations have just taken them away from home. I believe my meditation and my daily gratitudes have helped my mind shift to a more positive outlook on my daughters being far away from home. Do I miss them? Every single day. But, I know they are where they need to be.

I still run my own business, which comes with its own set of stresses as well. However, I have a support team around me that helps me see the opportunities, instead of the challenges.

ACTION PLAN

There are hundreds of ways to help you decompress. The idea is to find the ones that work best for you. One way that everyone can help lower their cortisol, is to monitor the foods they eat. Nutrition is a huge factor in either increasing or decreasing your blood sugars. Remember, the increased cortisol > increased blood sugar > increased insulin > increased cortisol cycle.

You can go back to the mindset chapter and go through some of the tools you used there that helped you to be more positive. These same tools will help you relax as well. Let's also go back to how you think and talk to yourself. This will either increase or decrease your stress levels. If you have negative dialogue in your head, this will increase your cortisol. Remember also; what your mind thinks, your body will take action on.

Meditation and breathing techniques are another great way to reduce your stress. "It clears my head, creates a sense of calm over my body and I'm ready to take on whatever the day has to bring in just 10 minutes." -- Ann

She now finds that meditating early in the morning, before the rest of her family wakes up, is the best time and solution for her.

Ann is understanding the importance of staying calm in a stressful situation. But, the biggest lesson she has learned is the need to care for herself first, in order to take better care of her family. This is known as self-care.

Here is a beautiful quote by Eleanor Brown that says:

"Rest and self-care are so important. When you take time to replenish your spirit, it allows you to serve others from the overflow. You cannot serve from an empty vessel."

Self-care is not a selfish act, it's an opportunity to create your best self, through what most of us recognize as preventive medicine. By allowing yourself the best possible care, both mentally and physically, you become your best self. Then, you can give others your best self, too. How could that be selfish?

Which action steps will you take to reduce your stress?

5

Support

All three of our ladies needed guidance, structure, and accountability to help them to attain their goals. They needed a guide, someone to show them the roadmap of how to get to where they all wanted to be. They needed to not feel like they were doing this by themselves and they wanted to have fun while they were fulfilling their goals.

Sometimes asking for help is the bravest thing you can do. You are going to learn how to build a strong support system. Of course you can go it alone, but why would you when it's more fun and effective with an army behind you?

There are different aspects of a support team:

- Coaching or expertise
- Community
- Family and Friends

COACH

Athletes for years have been dependent on coaches to help them get to the next level. Today, when you want to improve something, you reach out to find answers from an expert in that specific field. Whether it is in business, home maintenance, financial planning, or physicians, etc.

Finding a coach to help you become a healthier version of yourself is no different. When you decide that you need a coach, it is important to make sure they have your best interest at heart, not their own agenda. That means the coach should be focused on your individual growth and goals. What is best for you and for your family.

They should be committed to your safety and developing a personalized roadmap just for you, not what has worked for them or any of their other clients.

A good coach will keep you motivated, even on the days when you are not your strongest. They will keep you accountable for your short and long term goals and keep you moving forward on your path.

Who needs a coach?

Quite frankly, everyone, I did! We all need a little coaching or improvement at some point in the journey. Here is why Jennifer, Ann and Susan all hired us to coach them.

Jennifer: felt very comfortable in a gym setting, because she did the same routine every day. She couldn't figure out why she wasn't losing weight, despite her efforts. After explaining to her how a smart training program works and what it looks like to eat a supportive nutrition plan, Jennifer was on the right path to dropping her 10 pounds for her class reunion and rocking her little black dress.

Ann: didn't know where to start, and other gyms she had walked into were big and intimidating.

She knew she needed not only help with her training program, but also her nutrition. After talking with us during her first sit down meeting, she felt safe, excited and knew she had found her new place.

Susan: had joint issues, her knees and her back were giving her problems more than ever. But she wanted an expert to come up with a plan to help her with more balance and strength and someone who would keep her safe, not make matters worse.

When searching for a coach, make sure they are certified or come highly recommended. The few reputable certifications I like are NSCA, NASM, ACSM, and ACE. I know there are many more and having a certification doesn't make you a great coach, but it's a good place to start. Make sure they ask you a lot of questions about your goals, past and present, medical conditions, nutrition, sleep, and stress. You also need to click with them, personality wise! If they don't ask you questions and just want to get started right away, find a new trainer.

COMMUNITY

Another way you can find support is through the community in which you train.

Here at Oxygen + Iron we pride ourselves on having a strong community. Our members are not only workout buddies, who help keep each other accountable and motivated during the training sessions, but they are friends outside the studio as well.

Our members don't call our studio a "gym." To them, it doesn't feel like the big box gyms they were accustomed to in the past. They feel welcomed and accepted here. They are not intimidated by how they look or what they wear or where they are in their own fitness journey. Our members know when each other are on vacation or sick. They know their spouses name and where they work. What their children's names are and what schools they attend. It feels like an extended family, and they never feel alone.

Our coaches may give our members guidance, but it is our members give each other the feeling of being part of something bigger—a team, tribe, circle or whatever you want to call it. Being part of a community helps you stay motivated and on your path.

FAMILY and FRIENDS

Another very important part of your support team will come from your family and friends. Your inner circle.

Generally speaking, those closest to us will usually have the most influence over us. As motivational speaker Jim Rohn states, *"You are the average of the five people you spend the most time with."* In other words, who you spend most of your time with can influence the person you may become, good or bad. When you are trying to change a habit, it is best to associate with like-minded people to help you make this change.

Being in a supportive environment will help you stay on track no matter the challenges ahead. My inner circle is tight, and to this day, they are my biggest supporters, as I am for them.

Many times you can influence your family and friends to join you with your journey, this only strengthens the ride. I would say about 90% of the men in our studio have joined because of their spouse or partner. It makes things much smoother and more fun if you have more of your tribe on board!

But what if you don't have the support of your family or friends?

Unfortunately, this does happen.

Have you ever heard of the crab theory?

It is a theory that describes a way of thinking, or you may have heard the phrase,

"if I can't have it, neither can you."

The metaphor refers to a pot of crabs. Individually, the crabs could easily escape from the pot, but instead, if one tries to get out, the other crabs in the pot will grab at it, as in a useless "king of the hill" competition, which prevents any of the crabs from escaping and ensures their collective demise.

The analogy in human behavior is that members of a group will attempt to "pull down" any member who achieves success beyond the others, out of conspiracy, envy, or competitive feelings.

If you feel like you are not getting the support from either your family or friends, just remember this is YOUR journey, not theirs. Find support from a coach or a studio with a great community.

6

Training

Did you know that sitting is the new smoking? According to a Mayo clinic doctor, prolonged sitting and a sedentary lifestyle increases the risk of developing heart disease, some cancers, and type 2 diabetes. Not to mention an increase in obesity.

Isn't that enough to get you out of your chair? Today's modern world has us sitting more than ever; at work, in our cars, and on the couch. It is wreaking havoc on our bodies. It's time to get up and move!

Where do you start? What do you do?

This is where the confusion begins. This is where I hear all the reasons why I shouldn't workout. It's boring. I will get bulky. I will be sore. I have a bad knee or a bad back. I do cardio (isn't that good enough?). I'm embarrassed or intimidated to go into the gym by myself. And, the list goes on....

I have solutions for all of those and more. You need a plan, a simple plan, but most of all you just need to MOVE more.

Before coming to our studio, Ann was nervous and embarrassed to go to the big box gym close to her home, because she had no idea what to do once she got inside the gym. She truly thought everyone who worked out there was super fit and knew exactly what they were doing.

We designed a well-balanced training program that she does 4 times a week, on most weeks. She trains with a coach once a week and workouts with her friends in class the other 3 days. Her coach explained why she was doing each exercise as well as how it should be done correctly. Ann is now confident enough in her knowledge and abilities that, when she goes on vacation, she has no qualms about walking into the hotel gym.

ACTION PLAN

Where to start.

In order to be successful, you must go back to your WHY and to your GOALS. Your training program needs to be designed with you in mind. The plan must take into consideration your whys, needs, goals, time schedule, and likes and dislikes in order for you to become your best self.

Here are some guidelines on how we create a great training program at our studio.

When you are looking for a training program, make sure you follow these guidelines.

SAFETY

Above all else, safety comes first at our studio, whether it's during a class or a private training session. When you are in a new gym, it is the coach's job to keep you safe. They must make certain you are doing the exercises correctly and that the space around you is safe at all times. Your program should be well designed specifically for you. There may be exercises that you can't do at the moment, due to an old injury or some muscle stiffness that prohibits your body from going through the movement properly. A great coach will either modify or exchange that exercise for something that is more suitable for you.

At times you may find that you get a little competitive when in a group class setting, but try not to get pulled into the vortex. Your workout is based off your abilities, fitness level, and movement patterns. You don't want to be in an environment where you are competing against the other members there, to prove you are fit, or to need to gain another badge. Pushing yourself is one thing, pushing yourself to the point you feel like throwing up, or worse, getting injured is just not safe.

Susan told us that she couldn't do squats, because it made her knees hurt. Though her knees hurt her every day, and her doctor told her to strengthen the muscles around her knees. She was convinced that doing squats or lunges would make them worse. We explained to her how the muscles worked and showed her how to do a squat correctly.

Today, Susan is doing variations of squats, lunges and deadlifts and best of all, her knees have stopped hurting every day.

WARM UP

Most people know they NEED to do a warm-up or "stretch" before they workout, but most don't think it's important. And they tend to skip it. THIS IS A MISTAKE!

Studies have shown that warming up and stretching improves your physical performance and prevents injuries—especially a warm-up that increases your body temperature and uses similar movements as in your training program.

At our studio, we do different types of movements that will increase your core body temperature and increase your mobility. We call this our RAMP which stands for:

Range of motion—these are stretching and/or mobility type exercises.

Activation—these are exercises for the muscles around the hips and shoulder blades.

Movement Preparation—dynamic stretching and movements that take the body through multiple planes of motion.

If you take your warm up or RAMP seriously, you will be better prepared for the best training session possible. And it will help to keep your body healthier and help reduce injuries in the process.

"I felt like an old lady, my knees and back hurt all the time. My shoulders were beginning to round forward and I had trouble getting up off the floor," Susan remembered. "Now, I stand tall with my shoulders back and can easily touch my toes."

STRENGTH TRAINING

What is the biggest misconception about training for women?

That doing more cardiovascular training is the best way to get in shape, to change your body or to be fit. I'm here to set the record straight; strength training, or resistance training, is the only way (besides nutrition of course) to transform your body the way that you want it to look, feel and move. Not by cardio, not running, spin class, kickboxing, treadmill or the elliptical. Your body must push against resistance to change.

As you age, you lose more muscle mass and gain more body fat. As women, we produce less testosterone in our bodies, which makes it harder for us to gain muscle. When you have less muscle that means performing everyday activities will begin to get much harder to do. This is why I make sure every woman is doing some sort of strength training program, regardless of her age or fitness level.

The added benefit of having more muscle mass, is that it requires more calories to maintain basic body functions while at rest, which is called your Resting Metabolic Rate. This means your metabolism increases and who doesn't want a faster metabolism as you age?

There are many different styles of strength training and tools you can use, like your own bodyweight, dumbbells, kettlebells, sandbags, bands and more. At the studio, we use all of these tools to design our metabolic resistance training classes—which is a fancy name for strength circuit training. These classes are quick, but effective, only lasting 30 minutes. You will burn maximum calories and help boost your metabolism.

This type of training will create what is called an "after-burn"—meaning you will continue to burn calories after the session for 24-48 hours. Unlike cardio where the burning process stops after you finish exercising. Talk about getting a big bang for your buck. You will add muscle tone while burning fat at the same time.

Who has time for 2-hour training sessions in the gym? Not me.

Before Jennifer came to us, she was exercising 30 minutes on the treadmill, doing weight machines and then finishing it off with another 30 minutes on the elliptical. She couldn't understand why her body never changed. In fact, she was gaining weight each year instead of losing or maintaining. After we explained the benefits of the after-burn and a proper strength training program (not some random machines), she is now losing her muffin top and has definition in her arms.

The only time she works out for an hour now is when she meets her girlfriends for a hike.

CARDIO

"I must do more cardio." That is probably the phrase I hear most from women getting back into fitness or wanting fat loss. This could not be further from the truth. The days of running on a treadmill, pounding away on the elliptical, or endless hours in spin class are over. Well, at least they should be over!

These types of exercises won't help you with fat loss in the long term and they are very repetitive, which leads to various overuse injuries. Did you know that 75% of runners develop some type of injury? 75%. That doesn't sound like a safe way to lose fat to me. Now, I'm not saying you can't run or shouldn't run. I know a LOT of people run for many reasons. But if your goal is fat loss, running should not be your number one priority.

Okay, I could go on and on about running, but for now let's just say—running is not the best option for fat loss. Neither is a spin class, the elliptical or any type of long steady state cardio. Aerobic or steady state cardio do have their place in the fitness world, but it would be the last element I would integrate into a training program. I would suggest some type of interval training. Interval training is any exercise that alternates between high intensity and low intensity recovery periods, think sprints or old fashion suicides.

The high intensity would be as hard as you can go for a set amount of time, followed by either rest or lower intensity activity. This type of training has been proven to burn more calories than steady state cardio, over a shorter period of time. In other words, you don't have to spend hours on the treadmill to gain the same benefits as interval training.

Back to being more efficient and effective, interval training will put your body in the after-burn state, too. Incorporating interval training into your training program is just another tool to help you lose fat, if that is one of your goals. If you still need or want to do aerobic exercise, I would suggest that you do it after your intervals.

HAVE FUN

Make sure the workout is fun! There is nothing worse than doing something you dread every day. This will lead to boredom, misery and no training. Training shouldn't be torturous either. I'm not suggesting that all my members like burpees or other exercises that we do in our group training classes, but they do love being in class with their friends. They love the music (most of the time) and they love how they feel when finished. Make sure you find somewhere that has an inviting environment, like we have at our studio. Find a place where you feel comfortable and know that the coaches are there to help you. Maybe even try working out with a buddy, like Susan did, it will definitely make it more fun. Plus, you will keep each other more accountable.

STEPS TO A GREAT FAT LOSS PROGRAM

To get the most out of your training program for fat loss, here is the hierarchy we use at the studio. Choose which elements according to how much time you realistically have each week:

1. Always use strength training. This should be part of your plan no matter how much time you have. If you only have an hour 3 days a week, make it strength training.

Three days a week for strength training is ideal, make sure you have one day of rest between each training session. You don't want to go back to back days with this. Your body needs time to recover.

2. Incorporate some type of interval training. We suggest 2-3 times per week. These sessions would be great on your off days of strength training.

3. Long steady state cardio. If you still have more time in your schedule, by all means do some type of cardio. But only if you have the time and most of all if you enjoy the activity. Don't do it just to do it. A rest day would be more beneficial to you and your body. But I do understand some women need this mostly for their minds. Then go for it!

Mobility, strength training and interval training are not the only pieces to the puzzle of a smart training program. You must know how and when to recover. Just as important as strength training is to your muscles, recovery is important to your entire body.

RECOVERY

Most people think recovery has to do with your off training days or doing some type of stretching program like yoga. These are a few tools you may use, but recovery is so much more than just trying to get rid of yesterday's muscle soreness. Both your body and your brain need to recover daily. Burning the candle at both ends is not a badge of honor, it is a disaster waiting to happen.

When your body recovers, it helps you reduce your stress. Many of the same tools you use for stress management can be used for recovery too. Meditation, massage, Epsom salt baths, reading, journaling, getting outside and, most importantly, sleep.

Once Ann got on the right path and she discovered the tools to help her decompress, she finally started seeing the results she was looking for. She does her meditation in the morning, then comes to the studio for her workouts (which includes a proper warm up) to help with her hips and back tightness. She is eating supportive meals. And, she ends her evening, either reading or taking an Epsom salt bath. She is averaging around 7.5 - 8 hours of sleep a night which is giving her more energy.

Ann still has to be in the car all afternoon with her kids and has all the other responsibilities as before, but by making a few tweaks in her day and making herself a priority, she feels less stressed and her body and mind feel more relaxed.

"I feel like I have more energy during the day and I'm not completely exhausted at the end of the night, not to mention, my family says I'm more pleasant to me around."

You also need a day off to allow your body to truly recover, especially after your strength days. On these days of rest, your muscles are repairing and replenishing themselves. Recovery also helps to rebuild and restore many of your other systems to get ready for the next day.

Your mind needs a break from the day to day stresses as well. You need time away from your pressures and the many noises you live amongst—inside and outside your head. You also need to get away from indoor lighting, and the many screens you may look at all day long is harmful to your eyes.

The most effective and easiest way to recover, is by getting more sleep. It is recommended that adults should get somewhere between 7-9 hours of restful sleep a night. Today, most of us are getting less than 6! Which means you start your next day at a disadvantage. When this pattern continues day after day, you start to see problems.

You may experience a foggy brain. Or your immune system gets compromised and you become sick all the time. Or, you may start to gain weight and even begin to feel depressed.

Getting adequate sleep every night can be tricky with your busy lifestyle. Again going back to earlier in the book, when you are over stressed and don't self-manage well, your sleep is usually the first thing that takes the hit. You try to finish everything on your to do list. And, before you realize it, it's midnight and you have to up by 6 am the next morning.

Once this cycle starts and you keep losing sleep, your metabolism will get thrown off. This means your blood sugar and insulin elevate, which causes you to gain weight. More on this in the nutrition chapter, but you get the picture.

Here are a few simple tools to help you sleep like a baby:

- A cool and dark room
- No screens 30 minutes prior to bedtime
- No caffeine after 2 pm
- Take a bath before bed
- Read a book
- Drink some tea (Chamomile)
- Try journaling

Some days you don't need a complete rest from training, which is called an active recovery day. Active recovery, is when you do some type of cross-training at a lower intensity in order to just get blood flowing to your muscles to help them recover. You could go play tennis, take a walk, play at the playground with your kids, all of these can be active rest.

My favorite type of active rest is hiking. Here in Richmond we have extensive trails in our park system around the James River. I can literally be 10 minutes from downtown and feel like I am deep in the woods. Hiking these trails does more for me mentally than any meditation session could do. I walk through the woods with all senses on high alert, smelling the vegetation, hearing the birds, listening mostly for cardinals, feeling the ground beneath my feet, and taking in all the sights—from other hikers to walkers to bikers. Not to mention a few sightings of wildlife, like raccoons, deer, woodpeckers and of course snakes! An hour on the trail and I am recharged for the next couple of days and wanting to go back for more.

Don't underestimate the power of recovery. It doesn't make you weak. What it does do is make you a smart for actually listening to your body and doing what's best for you.

Here are the tools again, that will help you recover on your days off. Find the ones that work the best for you:

- Self-management with your time
- Getting adequate sleep
- Exercise, yoga, walking
- Meditate
- Journaling
- Daily gratitudes
- Positive self-talk
- Epsom salt bath
- Massage

7

Nutrition

This may be the hardest area for most women to accomplish. Food, at times, is either your enemy or your friend depending on the circumstance. You may have tried this diet or that diet, none of which have been successful long term. We all have to eat, but what you eat can either help you or harm you.

We truly are what we eat. You need to eat according to what your body needs in order to stay healthy. This is called supportive nutrition. For you to become your best self, you need to get away from the Standard American Diet (SAD) of processed foods and sugar and start fueling your body with the nutrients it needs, wants and craves.

I'm sure you have heard the saying before that "you can't out train a bad diet" and this is absolutely true. You could have the best training program in the world, but if you don't support it with healthy nutrition you will never see the results you are looking for. If that's not enough, poor nutrition will make you sick, fat, and tired. Who wants that?

So, where do you start?

To be honest, there is no magic bullet when it comes to nutrition. I am going to make it as simple as I can. I could go deep and explain exactly what you need to eat, how much, and how often, but it would be different for everyone.

Nutrition is very personal. What works for one person may not work for the next. So, what I am going to give you are simple parameters to work with instead.

The first thing I ask my members to do is to write in a food journal. This is not meant in any way to judge what they are eating, but it gives me and their coaches a quick snapshot of how and what they eat. It will help us figure out where we need to start with them nutrition-wise.

When a member gets off track with their nutrition, a food journal is the first thing I ask them to do again. It is a great tool for both the coach and for the member. This awareness of what they are eating will, many times, be enough to get them back on track. If you have never done a food journal before, I suggest you try it for 3 days. Write down EVERYTHING you eat or drink. I highly recommend you do it, as painful as it may seem—it's worth it. Find the daily food journal at the back of the book.

WHAT TO EAT

When it comes to nutrition, I try to make it as simple as eating REAL FOOD—meaning foods that are basically single ingredient foods—not processed or manufactured. Lean proteins, vegetables, fruits, and healthy fats.

LEAN PROTEINS

Proteins is used as a main source of energy. It is an essential building block for muscle, bones, cartilage, skin and blood—along with transporting enzymes, vitamins and hormones. Here are a few examples of high quality protein that you should be eating at every meal:

Organic grass fed beef and bison
Organic free range chickens and eggs
Wild caught fish and seafood
Organic pasture raised pig
Whey protein powder
Cheese and yogurt.

If you are a vegetarian, you still need protein. Try these plant based sources of protein:

Spinach

Sun-dried tomatoes

Artichokes

Peas

Beans

Lentils

Nuts and seeds

VEGETABLES

Vegetable are considered a complex carbohydrate. Their main purpose is also to produce energy for the body. Veggies are high in fiber, taking the body a longer time to break down and use for energy—thus making it harder to store as fat. I'm sure you know what vegetables are, but here are a few of my favorites: spinach, broccoli, squash, avocado, peppers, asparagus, and Brussels sprouts.

Just like the lean proteins you need to have vegetables at each meal.

HEALTHY FATS

Believe it or not, your body need fat. Now let me get this out of the way, fat does not make you fat and good fat will not increase your cholesterol levels. I know this is all very confusing, so let me make it as simple as possible.

There are good fats and bad fats. Here are the bad fats: trans-fat. Anything labeled partially hydrogenated oil is a trans-fat and should be avoided. It is mostly artificial and increases your LDL and raises your HDL the so-called good cholesterol.

Here are some good fats and high fat foods you can use for supportive nutrition:

Avocados
Seeds and nuts and their butters
Olives and olive oil
Flaxseed
Eggs
Salmon
Tofu.

You should be looking to include healthy fats at least 1-2 times per day.

STARCHY CARBOHYDRATES

This is where food gets tricky. Starchy carbs are food such as rice, pasta, breads and potatoes. While your body uses these carbs for energy or fuel, a lot of these items can cause inflammation and wreak havoc on your gut. It takes a lot of trial and error on your part when it comes to which starchy carbohydrates are right for your body.

But if you know which ones your body can tolerate, you can eat them—but use sparingly. That goes for fruit too. Both starchy carbs and fruit, are best to eat after you workout, to allow the body to use them to refuel your muscles.

HOW MUCH TO EAT

The easiest way to figure out how much real food you should be eating is to picture a dinner plate divided into sections. One for lean proteins, one for vegetables, one for healthy fats and maybe one for starchy carbohydrates.   If your plate contains all 3-4 of these items, you are now eating a supportive nutritional diet and real food.

ACTION STEPS

There is so much more to nutrition then what I have discussed so far. Remember these tips are just a starting point. If you need more information or direction, you can ask your coach. But remember a fitness coach cannot design exact meal plans without being a registered dietitian. However, most of us know enough about nutrition to get people on the right track.

The biggest thing is to try not to make nutrition so complicated, keep it simple. Here's how:

- eat lean protein and veggies at every meal
- include healthy fats at least 1-2 times per day

- have fruits and starchy carbs after training.
- EAT REAL FOOD!
- food journal

Some other frequently asked questions about nutrition are:

1- What can I drink?

2- Do I have to give up my wine?

3 -Should I take supplements?

4- How much water should I be drinking per day?

SUPPLEMENTS

Let's start with the question of supplements, since we just finished with food. Ideally, you should get all our nutrients from your food. This shouldn't be a big problem if you are eating organically and eating real food. However, I am also realistic. There are times when you don't eat as clean as you should. So, to be safe, I would suggest a good whole food multi-vitamin. I also like to add two more vitamins to my list— vitamin D and fish oil for Omega 3's. My suggestion is either ask your primary care doctor or your pharmacist for the correct dosage for you.

WATER

Next, let's move on to what should I be drinking? My first answer will always be water. Your body are primarily made up of water. Your body requires about half your bodyweight in ounces of water per day. The average American woman weighs roughly 166 pounds, so that means she should be drinking about 83 ounces of water per day.

Obviously, you don't want to drink 83 ounces at one sitting, spread it out throughout the day and you shouldn't have trouble getting it in. Start your day off with a tall glass of water. Carry around a water bottle all day, keep refilling it, this will help you to remember to DRINK YOUR WATER! Please stick with pure water, if you need to flavor your water, use fruits and veggies, like berries, citrus and cucumbers.

TEAS, SODA and COFFEE

Other liquids that are okay to drink would be teas and coffee. It is not ideal to use caffeinated drinks for your afternoon pick me ups, limit your caffeine consumption after 2 pm, this way it won't interrupt your much needed sleep.

Fruit juices are loaded with sugar, though the sugar is real. To your body, sugar is sugar, it doesn't know the difference—and your body doesn't need sugar, ever! This brings us to soda, diet or not, it's a flat out NO. In a 12 oz. can of Coke there is 39 grams of sugar—THIRTY-NINE! I have no words. Diet sodas are not any better with their artificial sweeteners, I will save the debate about the horrors of soda for another book.

But, the answer is still no. Not one a day, not any. Drinking soda and smoking is where I put my foot down. If you could see me, my hands would be on my hips, too.

ALCOHOL

Let's talk alcohol. Ah, the glass of wine at the end of the day to unwind. Sounds good in theory, but your body won't like it and here is why. Alcohol temporarily stops your body from burning fat. Your metabolic system stops its normal functioning to get rid of the alcohol. So, whatever you recently ate, will get stored as fat. This is better known as a beer gut!

I'm not saying don't drink alcohol, that's a personal choice. I'm just giving you the reality of how your body reacts to it. Remember moderation is always the key. I will be explaining more about moderation in the next chapter.

Again this isn't a complete guide on nutrition, but some good guidelines to help you start creating healthier eating habits.

Here is a quick recap:

- Eat Lean Proteins at each meal
- Eat Veggies at each meal

- Eat Fruits and Complex Carbs sparingly and preferably after your training
- Drink ½ your body weight in water each day
- Take a multivitamin, Vitamin D and fish oil every day
- Use in moderation: coffee, teas and alcohol
- Start with a food journal

8

Lifestyle

What does it actually mean to live a healthy lifestyle?

The *World Health Organization* defines HEALTH as "a complete state of mental, physical and social well-being not merely the absence of disease."

And *Wikipedia* defines a LIFESTYLE as "a way a person lives."

We could say that healthy living are the steps, actions and strategies one puts in place to achieve optimum health. Over the past few chapters, we have talked about these steps and actions you can take to help you live a healthier lifestyle. All aspects of your life, physical, emotional, and spiritual must work in harmony to create this well balanced healthy life.

Being active and living a healthy lifestyle will add quality years to your life. You will not only look better, move better, but you will feel better as you age. If you put it in the perspective that health is not a luxury and that self-care—both physically and mentally should be your number one daily priority- you will attain the goal of having a healthy lifestyle.

It really is simple. You can put in the time now, with the supportive nutrition, daily exercise, and reduction in stress. Or, you can pay later in medical bills or worse yet—your life. It all comes down to choices. This is a lifelong process, there is no quick fix or magic bullet. It is basically being consistent with your choices day after day. It's about moderation, like I talked about with drinking alcohol. Yes, you can have a glass of wine, and no you can't have one or two every night. Or you need to workout most days. No, you don't have to push yourself so hard that you get injured. But, don't beat yourself up either if you miss a day working out. Listen to your body, not your head, because your head will tell you to stay on the sofa. Try giving yourself a goal of not missing two workouts in a row.

You will have obstacles, challenges, and distractions thrown at you all of your life. That won't change. Living a healthy lifestyle is the sum total of all your choices. Ask yourself is this going to be an opportunity to eat well before the birthday party, and then maybe have that piece of cake. But tomorrow, it's back to eating healthy with no guilt. Or when you do go on vacation or travel for work, you get right back to your training program when you return home. Or better yet, you workout while you are away!

For me, living a healthy life means living within the 80/20 rule of life. Which means I make the majority (80%) of my choices healthy ones and the rest (20%) not quite as healthy. If I spend the majority of the time making the right decisions, then I can truly enjoy the 20% and still see the results I'm looking for.

This also means you don't have to be perfect. Nobody is perfect. The 80/20 rule allows you to live and play and still be healthy. If there are times when you need to reign it back in, especially your nutrition, because you have gotten off track, try 90/10 for a few weeks until you get back. The point is, you are in control of your destiny. You get to choose whether you want to live a healthy lifestyle or not.

Remember our three ladies and their SMART goals?

All very realistic and all following the 80/20 rule of life. They have learned the value in living their lives this way.

JENNIFER- rocked her reunion and lost her 10 pounds, plus 4 more. She continues to workout at the studio at least 4 times per week and has even recruited her best friend to join her in our metabolic resistance training classes.

"I feel energized and really good about myself, I eat differently, so clean, it has become routine now. I have learned the importance of meal planning and having a routine and planning ahead. 14 pounds and several inches gone! The muffin top is gone, too! I have gotten more fit and stronger, I'm at my best fitness level ever.

Being part of a group is a lot of fun and we all have similar goals which makes the workouts better. You need to make the commitment to yourself, it's worth it" –Jennifer

ANN - still meditates daily and has started to journal every morning too. She is still training hard and has picked up another day of personal coaching, she hasn't hit her goal weight yet, but she has dropped 2 pant sizes. She feels better than ever, and she enjoys her family walks.

"I was excited about losing body fat. I have not lost all my weight yet. I learned how to be more mindful in what I ate and my daily activities, whether it's gratitude or having more energy. I like being more mindful. The experience in a class environment is awesome, where you are surrounded by the same people—it feels like a family. The coaches make it very personalized for you. I feel like I am always getting the attention that I need, in the good way, and it's FUN." –Ann

SUSAN -feels 10 years younger than the day she stepped into the studio. She is more mobile and feels like her balance is better. She no longer uses the small weights in the class and feels stronger than ever before. She is even wearing sleeveless shirts now to show off her arms. Susan and her husband are going on a cross country road trip next year to hike in 4 different states.

"I feel stronger. I even bounce up and down the stairs, I feel like the Energizer bunny. I'm having so much fun and we are having fun in the training sessions. The personal attention, support and fun have made the biggest difference for me."—Susan

Living a healthy lifestyle isn't just about training and nutrition. We have talked about the importance of mindset, having a strong support team, stress management and recovery—all of which is based around your why and your goals. Like our motto at my studio says, "it's not just a workout, it's a LIFESTYLE!"

So what do you do with the other time you have that doesn't revolve around your goals?

That's called living! Living an active healthy life.

Do things you love, with the most important people in your lives.

This is where the magic is!

Stay present, get off your phones, computers and video games.

Pull yourself off the sofa, away from your desk, and start living.

Start a new hobby, call an old friend, take your dog for a walk and like it, connect with people and nature.

You will be amazed how much better you will feel. Your whole life feels structured, organized, stressed and chaotic. Take some time to get outside and just breathe.

GO OUTSIDE

Ever since I was a little girl, I felt most at home being outside. Either riding my bike, playing hide-and-go-seek with the neighborhood kids, or walking in the woods looking for adventures. Today, I don't play hide-and-go-seek much anymore, but I still ride my bike and walk in the woods. It brings me back to center, to a place of calm that I can't get anywhere else.

There is plenty of research to back up those same feelings of calm. Studies have shown that being outside is not only good for you mentally, but physically as well. We tend to be more active when we are outside. When you are outside you can get a healthy dose of Vitamin D, which is needed for bone and cell growth. It helps with inflammation reduction, and neuromuscular and immune function. It can help lower your heart rate and improve your sleep. There are an unlimited amount of reasons to get outside.

You don't have to be in the woods to gain the benefits of being outside. Go for a walk after dinner, ride your bike to the store, play with your kids on the playground—actually play with them—play tennis or golf or meditate outside. Make one of your training sessions outdoors. The list is endless.

OTHER WAYS TO STAY ACTIVE

There are other ways to stay active besides being outside:

- park farther away from an entrance
- take the stairs instead of the elevator
- bike to work
- garden
- stand up and walk around while you are on the phone.

Living a healthy lifestyle isn't rocket science, but it takes some work. Anything worth having, takes work!

We live in a world of instant gratification and quick fixes. We want everything to be easy and delivered to our doorstep. To maintain a healthy lifestyle, it requires a lifelong journey with no finish line. You need to put in the work, be a good role model for your children, and for yourself.

Did you know that right now we are in an era where our children may not live as long as we do? Which is a scary thought. All these years we've increased our life expectancy and we have all this technology and knowledge and now we're starting to go in the opposite direction. Just because we are making poor choices, in both our movement and nutrition. You need to be healthy for you, your kids, and for the next generation.

We all have struggles and we all have setbacks. No one person is busier or more important than another. This is the common tie that binds us. You have to figure out how to make the time and the effort to become healthy and be your best self. Make yourself a priority. Taking care of you doesn't mean you are selfish, it means that you are smart enough to know that you can't help others if you don't take care of yourself first.

WE ARE NOT DONE!

Bonus Materials

Finding Your Why Worksheet

If you change NOTHING about your current lifestyle, what does one year from now look like to you?

How will you look?

How will you feel?

Now, imagine yourself taking action; you are more active, eating healthy foods, taking time for yourself, feeling less stressed and all around feeling happier about who you are.

How do you look now?

How do you feel now?

S.M.A.R.T. Goals Worksheet

Specific: (Goals should be written simply and clearly define what you are going to do.)

Specific is the What, Why, and How?

Measurable: (Goals should be measurable so that you have proof that you have accomplished the goal. i.e., train 4 x per week, meditate every morning, eat protein for breakfast every day) What gets measured, gets done!

Achievable: Goals should be achievable; they should stretch you slightly so you feel challenged, but attainable so that you can achieve them.

What are your short term goals? What are your long term goals?

Relevant: activities that make sense with entire goal. List how your daily activities will be realistic towards achieving your specific goals.

Time-sensitive: Goals should be linked to a timeframe that creates a practical sense of urgency. Without such tension, the goal is unlikely to produce a relevant outcome.

What does your timeline look like?

Training

Quick 10-minute burst
BURST A
20 seconds work, 10 seconds rest x 8 rounds
High Knees
Jumping Jacks
Rest 1 minute and REPEAT circuit

BURST B
20 seconds work, 10 seconds rest x 8 rounds
Mountain Climbers
Skaters
Rest 1 minute and REPEAT circuit

A/B STRENGTH sample
Do workout A on day 1, workout B on day 2, workout A on day 3. Must have one complete day's rest in between workouts.

Workout A
1)Plank 3 x for 30 seconds, with 30 seconds rest after each

2A) Goblet Squat
2B) Alternating Dumbbell Arm Row

3 sets of each superset. Perform exercise 2A for 12 reps, followed by 12 reps of exercise 2B with no rest. Rest 60 seconds after each superset.

Move on to next superset

3A) Sumo Dumbbell Deadlift
3B) Push Ups
3 sets of each superset. Perform exercise 3A for 12 reps, followed by 12 reps of exercise 3B with no rest. Rest 60 seconds after each superset.

Workout B
1)Bicycle crunch 3 sets of 12 reps, with 30 seconds rest after each

2A) Reverse Lunge (each leg)
2B) Upright Row

3 sets of each superset. Perform exercise 2A for 12 reps, followed by 12 reps of exercise 2B with no rest. Rest 60 seconds after each superset.

Move on to next superset

3A) Floor Bridge
3B) Push Up

3 sets of each superset. Perform exercise 3A for 12 reps, followed by 12 reps of exercise 3B with no rest. Rest 30 seconds after each superset.

If you don't live in the Richmond, VA area, but would like a training program designed specifically for you, please email me at linda@oxygenandiron.com. We do provide online training.

Supportive Nutrition
Recommended Food Sources

Proteins

Lean Ground Beef (90% of leaner)
Flank Steak
Sirloin Steak
Beef Filet/Tenderloin
Round
Chicken Breast
Turkey Breast
Ground Turkey Breast
Chicken Sausages*
Eggs* (3 eggs = 1 serving)
Egg Whites (1/2 cup = 1 serving)
Fish
Shrimp
Salmon*
Pork Tenderloin
Boneless Pork Chops
Boneless Pork Loin
Bison
Cottage Cheese (low- or non-fat)
Greek Yogurt (non-fat)
Protein Powder (whey or casein)

*includes 1 serving of fat as well
Carbohydrates

Most Fruits
Rice
White Potatoes
Sweet Potatoes
Oatmeal
Quinoa
Tortilla (1 med = 1 serving)
Beans
Pumpkin
Corn
Spaghetti or Butternut Squash

Vegetables

Spinach
Broccoli
Cauliflower
Peppers
Onion
Tomato
Cucumbers
Zucchini
Yellow Squash
Asparagus
Brussel Sprouts
Green Beans
Peas
Carrots
Artichoke

Eggplant

Celery

Kale

Romaine

Cabbage

Bok Choy

Watercress

Radishes

Turnip

Parsley

Shallots

Sauerkraut

Mushrooms

Collards

Salsa

Fats

Extra Virgin Olive Oil

Coconut Oil

Nut Butters (almond, cashew, peanut)

Raw mixed nuts

Avocado

Flax meal

Butter (grass fed if possible)

Ghee

Cheeses

Pumpkin Seeds

Sunflower seeds

Chia Seeds

If you would like more information about supportive nutrition, please email me at linda@oxygenandiron.com.

Daily Food Journal

Date:_____

Time:
Food/Drink Amount:
Water (16oz per block):
Exercise:
Amount of Time:
Active Rest:
Supplements/Greens Post Workout Shake:
Sleep in Hours:

What is your WIN Today?
How do I Feel Today?

Daily Gratitude's
1.
2.
3.

Did You Meditation/Prayers Today?   How Long?

About the

Author

Linda's WHY:

I always knew I wanted to do something with physical fitness or health and wellness. I began helping people in health clubs over 30 years ago. Back then, it was more or less all about the workouts and making people look better, feel better, and making sure that they were training correctly. As I moved on through my career, it has been more about making people move more and feel stronger, both mentally and physically, just helping them feel better overall.

I coached for a long time in a big box gym. As I trained clients, I was constantly worrying about making my quota. This was difficult for me morally, because it wasn't my philosophy on how to help someone reach their overall goals. Sure I was giving them quality training and helping them attain their "fitness" goals, but it was harder to help them achieve all of their health and wellness goals.

I knew that there was a better solution for people and I knew that I could provide that solution. So, I decided to open my own studio. I had no idea what I was getting into business-wise. But I knew I was a good coach. I knew I could help my clients accomplish all of their goals.

Here is why I started my own studio and personal training business:

I didn't feel like my clients were getting what they need from the big box gym. I opened my studio hoping to change that, I started out with my vision to have a better place to workout for my clients. I opened this beautiful boutique style studio, hoping that would create a better atmosphere during our coaching sessions. My "why" has evolved since day one. Now that we have been here 9 years and running, I see our vision as not being in the workout or training business, but in the business of creating healthier lifestyles for busy people. Simply put, whether it's through training, mindset, nutrition, or an overall lifestyle balance, we empower women to become their best self. Our tagline is "It's not just a workout, it's a lifestyle" and that's what we have evolved into. A small beautiful boutique style studio, yes, but it's more about helping our clients change their lifestyle for the better!

Just like my clients who first start out on their new wellness journey, I encountered the ups and downs of owning my own business. It's a different skill set than coaching clients. It wasn't my wheel-house at first, but it became my passion to make sure that the doors stayed open and that I was providing the best service that I could for my members. I was determined to be a better solution than what was out there.

The reason for knowing your "why" is so important because we all go through ups and downs when you start on a new path. It's part of the process, it's what makes it so special when you succeed!

I know that living a healthy lifestyle has helped me move forward and stay strong—mentally and physically—throughout my life. I wanted and needed to help other women know that they can feel this way too, that it's hard, BUT WORTH IT.

My mission is to coach and guide these women to just do that. I sound a little like Wonder

Woman now, but you have a bit of superhero in you, you just need to bring her out!

My goal in writing this book is to share with you what I know works for my clients, as well as myself, and provide you with some tools that will get you started towards finding a healthier lifestyle, finding your inner superhero, and becoming your best self.

WE ARE NOT DONE.

If you live in the Richmond, VA area, please come visit me at my studio.

I would love to help you get started on becoming YOUR BEST SELF!

Oxygen + Iron Personal Training Studio
208 Heaths Way Road
Midlothian, VA 23114
804042301375

If you would like more information on any of the steps we went over in the book, please email me at linda@oxygenandiron.com

It's not just a workout, it's a LIFESTYLE!

Made in the USA
Columbia, SC
11 December 2017